One Effective Way to Hold a Deliberative Forum*

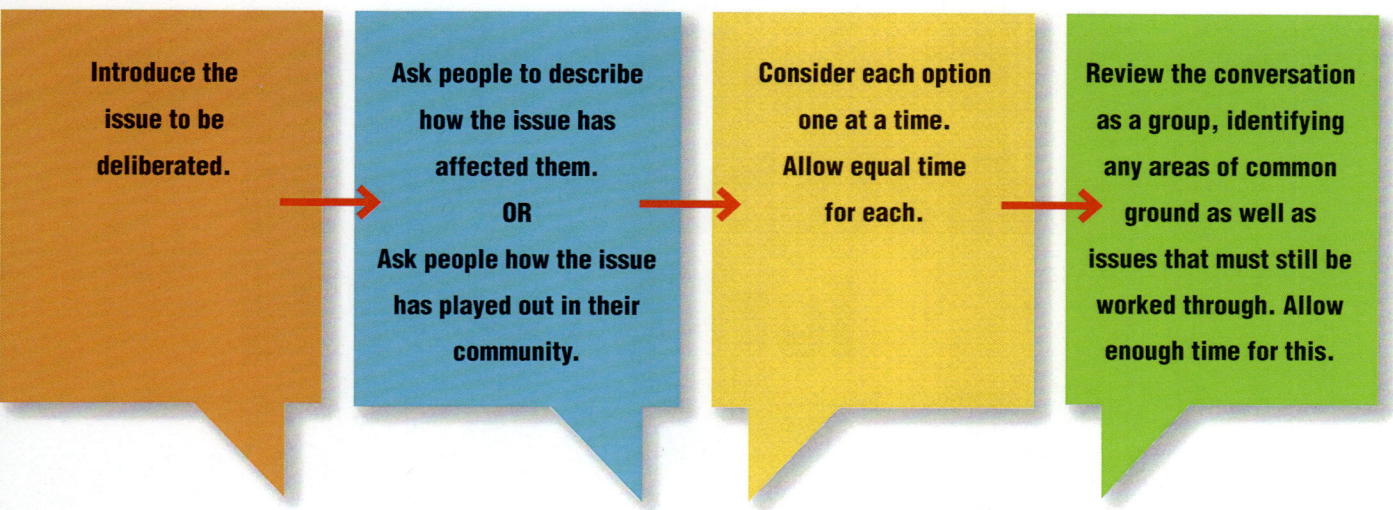

Introduce the issue to be deliberated.

Ask people to describe how the issue has affected them.
OR
Ask people how the issue has played out in their community.

Consider each option one at a time. Allow equal time for each.

Review the conversation as a group, identifying any areas of common ground as well as issues that must still be worked through. Allow enough time for this.

*This is not the only way to hold a forum. Some communities hold multiple forums.

Ground Rules for a Forum

Before the deliberation begins, it is important for participants to review guidelines for their discussion.

- Focus on the options.
- All options should be considered fairly.
- No one or two individuals dominate.
- Maintain an open and respectful atmosphere.
- Everyone is encouraged to participate.
- Listen to each other.

End of Life:

What Should We Do for Those Who Are Dying?

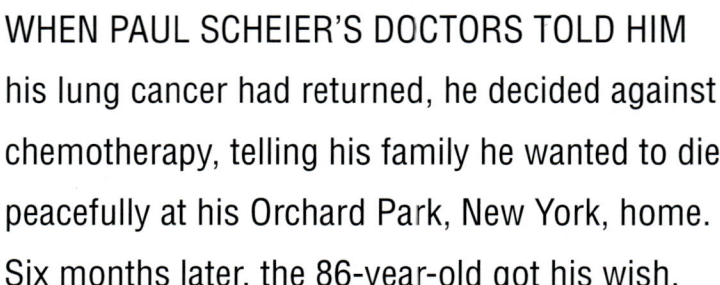

WHEN PAUL SCHEIER'S DOCTORS TOLD HIM his lung cancer had returned, he decided against chemotherapy, telling his family he wanted to die peacefully at his Orchard Park, New York, home. Six months later, the 86-year-old got his wish.

But the end for John Rehm, husband of radio talk show host Diane Rehm, wasn't so easy. Rehm, afflicted with Parkinson's Disease, was totally incapacitated when his request to hasten death was refused on moral and legal grounds. Maryland, where Rehm lived, is not one of five states where physician-assisted death is legal. Instead, Rehm refused water and food until he died of dehydration 10 days later.

What ought to be done at the end of life is both a personal and public decision. As our population ages, it is becoming a matter of great concern for the entire nation. Diseases that would have been death sentences a few decades ago are now often treatable.

"This is medicine's great problem currently," Dr. Lewis Goldfrank, director of Bellevue's emergency department told *60 Minutes.* "It will become greater and greater as the population ages. We'll save lives that no one could have imagined. But we prolong lives that people would have wished to abandon."

This guide explores end-of-life decisions and examines options and trade-offs inherent in this sensitive and universal issue. Medical advances make it more likely that we will care for relatives in their final days, facing decisions regarding their illnesses or death—as well as our own. Even those who never face such choices will pay for them through tax dollars and the cost of insurance premiums. And as more states consider passing "right-to-die" laws similar to the one that took effect in Oregon in 1997, this debate may become a local one.

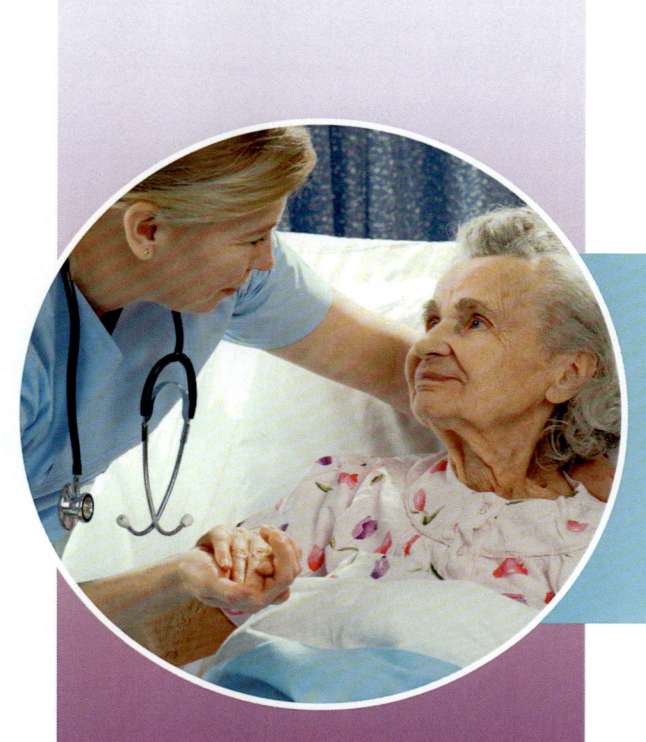

Adding to this is the fact that 100 million Americans have chronic diseases. Because of advances in medical science, many of these people can be kept alive through extremely painful and debilitating terminal stages of some of these illnesses. As a result, growing numbers of chronically ill people are asking for the right to take their own lives. These requests reflect their desire to die without further needless suffering.

In Oregon, for example, the majority of physician-assisted-death requests have come from those who have lost the ability to care for themselves. Not every request is carried through. Less than one percent of those who received "end of life" prescriptions actually used them. Clergy and ethicists are concerned that as more states pass laws that make it easier to die, the "right to die" may become a "duty to die," and that some lives will be valued more than others.

Should a dying young person be allowed to forego treatment that could extend his or her life? Should an active alcoholic receive a liver transplant that will cost the public thousands and deny a lifesaving organ to another? Is the public checkbook unlimited when it comes to preserving life at all costs? There are no easy answers.

The end of life is frequently the most expensive period of all: on average, Americans will spend five times the money on health care in their last year of life than in any one previous year. In 2011, Medicare spent $554 billion, of which 28 percent, or nearly $170 billion, was spent during the last six months of patients' lives. Public dollars are not limitless.

While more dying people are utilizing hospice services, the final days of most hospitalized patients are marked by aggressive treatments and runaway expenses, helping to make American medical care the most costly in the world. Some of the money spent on end-of-life care may ultimately not serve the patient well at all. Those dollars might be better spent helping people who have a better chance of recovery.

Under most circumstances, end-of-life decisions remain difficult and uncomfortable. A *Consumer Reports* survey found that 86 percent of those polled wanted to die at home.

But fewer than half of the respondents over age 65 had living wills detailing their dying wishes, leaving them at the mercy of hospitals and stressed-out families forced to decide on their behalf.

In 1990, the US Supreme Court affirmed an individual's "right to die." Later, in 1997, the court upheld New York and Washington state laws banning physician-assisted death, leaving it for individual states to decide their legality. These rulings established legal precedence for a national conversation.

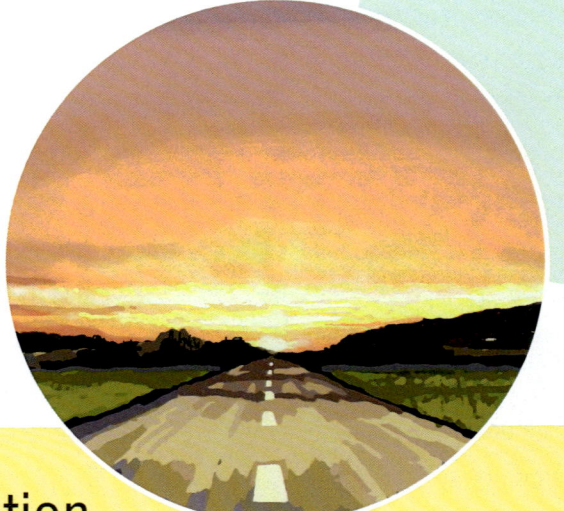

A **Framework** for Deliberation

This issue guide asks: What should society allow, and support, at the end of life? It presents three different ways of looking at the problem and suggests possible actions appropriate to each.

OPTION 1: **Maintain Quality of Life.** That means when continued efforts to keep terminally ill patients alive a few more days or weeks result in needless pain and suffering, life-support treatment should be discontinued. At that point, caregiving efforts should be devoted to keeping patients comfortable and pain free.

OPTION 2: **Preserve Life at All Costs.** Do everything we can to prevent death. This means sparing no expense to extend the lives of those who are sick. It should be difficult for doctors to give up on patients, and the end must not be brought about by deliberate medical neglect or intervention. Right-to-die laws must be repealed.

OPTION 3: **My Right, My Choice.** The freedoms we value so highly in choosing how we live should not be taken away from us at the end of our lives. People should have the right to end their own lives and to enlist their doctors in helping them to die when a terminal illness leaves nothing to look forward to but higher levels of pain and suffering.

Option 1:
Maintain Quality of Life

MEDICAL ADVANCES CAN KEEP PEOPLE ALIVE almost indefinitely. While these technologies work to increase life span, they sometimes do nothing beneficial for quality of life. A diminished quality of life is the reason most Americans would choose to die without further medical intervention.

One-third of US adults have written down their desires regarding end-of-life care. These advance directives (or living wills) tell doctors what to do in cases in which patients are unable to communicate their wishes. People may opt for cessation of treatment when they are chronically ill, in severe pain, or totally helpless.

Living pain free, with relative independence and with full mental capacity, is universally desired, according to this option. Improving and maintaining people's quality of life as long as possible should be our priority. But some treatments for the terminally ill are unlikely to prolong their lives for more than a few days or weeks while degrading their quality of life by causing more pain and suffering.

Avoid Painful and Debilitating Treatments

In this view, we should require doctors to use only the least invasive treatments for the terminally ill. Unnecessary medical procedures expose patients to physical ordeals and inflict both financial and emotional pain on them and their families.

"Avoiding unnecessary medical care is important because care that is not needed can be harmful to patients, and unnecessary care raises health-care costs for everyone," according to Richard J. Baron, MD, president and CEO of the ABIM Foundation, which advocates for advancing medical professionalism. Yet, in America, most doctors are paid by the services they give and the tests they order, often with little regard to cost. Left alone, the system itself rewards doctors for ordering more medical services, not fewer.

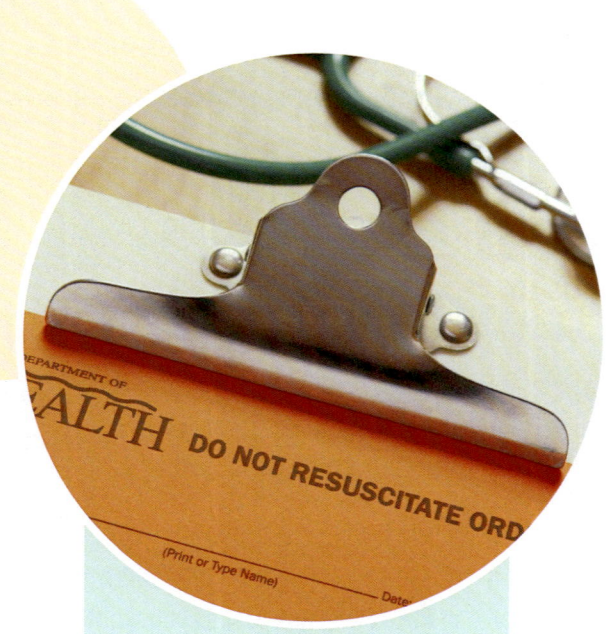

By restricting medical professionals from using certain painful, debilitating, and noncurative procedures, we can at least eliminate a major contributor to end-of-life suffering. Surgeries that do not cure, chemotherapy and radiation that create sicker patients, and unnecessary, invasive tests should only be used on those patients with a positive prognosis—those who are physically and emotionally strong enough to handle the side effects and results.

Standardize Quality-of-Life Definitions

We also need medical organizations to come up with a standard definition of "quality of life." Medical doctors should have a uniform understanding of "quality of life" and should be required to work within those boundaries. If a procedure would reduce a terminal patient's quality of life, it should not occur.

Many physicians struggle with making decisions about performing debilitating procedures. In the presence of a sick and dying patient, it can be difficult to convey the risks, especially when the patient insists that something be done.

"Post-diagnosis is a hard time to begin that conversation, because the patient is scared," Daniel Barocas, an assistant professor of urology at Vanderbilt University Medical Center, told *Scientific American*. "If you tell someone they have what they perceive as a lethal disease, they're going to seek treatment. This effort encourages discussions where doctors and patients can let data and evidence run the show a little instead of emotionality and fear."

Defining a good quality of life will not be easy. Setting standards will require a variety of voices. For most people the definition would include living pain-free, maintaining independence, and retaining a sound mind. But it will vary greatly among individuals and, in particular, among those with disabilities—some of whom live with conditions that make them less able to live independently or more prone to pain. For those people and for patients with serious illnesses, consideration will have to be given to matters of degree. In any case, in the last months or weeks of a terminal patient's life, this option holds that treatments that risk decreasing the present quality of life should not be undertaken.

Require Living Wills

Citizens should develop living wills. Doing so alleviates the emotional burden that loved ones experience when forced to make end-of-life decisions for a relative. Dying people should be strongly encouraged to develop living wills immediately following diagnosis.

The Caring Advocates organization has adopted a Plan Now, Die Later model for addressing end-of-life issues. They provide Advance Care Planning, a program designed to reduce suffering during the final stages of life. Surprisingly, it often leads people to choose to live longer.

Employers could require employees of a certain age to formulate a living will as part of their insurance policies. "What if, to be eligible for Medicare, you had to give someone power of attorney and sign a living will?" asked Ezra Klein in the *Washington Post*. This would surely cut down on much of the confusion and hardship faced by dying persons and their families. It could become a part of retirement planning to have a living will drawn up by the age of 45.

But some disagree. "The mere fact of putting words on paper can be distressing," Dr. Sean O'Mahoney, medical director of Montefiore Medical Center's palliative care services told the *New York Times*. He said he does not push hard for advance directives.

Reap What You Sow

This option holds that responsibility for quality of life lies as much with the individual as with his or her health-care practi-

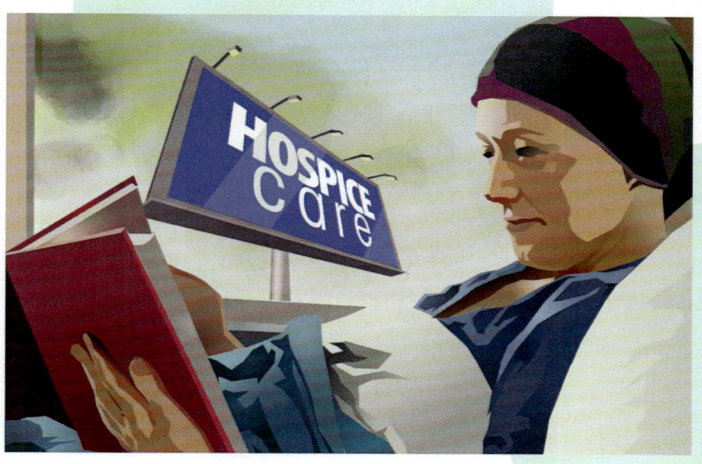

tioners. Dietary habits, lifestyle choices, and environmental pollutants contribute greatly to the leading causes of death in the United States. Right now, more than 70 percent of all deaths are caused by one or more chronic diseases. What if we could provide incentives for healthy living by either reward or punishment?

Unnecessary resources are spent to treat people who do things to destroy their own lives. Doctors respond to emergency room visits by those who undermine the very treatments they receive. Should doctors be forced to treat a person suffering from chronic obstructive pulmonary disease, which makes it hard to breathe, even if he insists on smoking a cigarette before getting into the ambulance? Should a person with liver failure be given access to treatment if she continues to consume alcohol?

An anonymous medical doctor, under the pseudonym Angienadia, lamented that half the patients in the intensive care unit "brought the condition upon themselves. I was being trained to undo what these people did to themselves, so that they can leave the hospital to do it some more. I wondered if we could ever draw a line, where we say enough is enough, where we say you do not get a second chance at life so that you can just kill yourself in the end."

By refusing to help those who destroy their own lives, we will encourage people to take better care of themselves and reduce the number of people suffering and dying from chronic diseases.

Invest More in Palliative Care

Palliative and hospice care have long ago proven to be beneficial for dying people. It improves the quality of life by decreasing pain, addressing depression, and by providing overall comfort for families and patients. In some cases, it even prolongs life.

Not only is palliative care good for the patient, but it saves money usually spent for hospitals and health-care practitioners. According to the University of Rochester Medical Center, palliative care intervention saved $630,000 in one year. "Whether you work in a 400-bed hospital or a 100-bed hospital, a palliative care program is likely to pay for itself in both reduced costs and increased patient satisfaction," said Raymond Hino, CEO of Mendocino Coast District Hospital in California, in a blog on FierceHealthcare.com.

In the long run, an investment in palliative care will improve end-of-life experiences. By reducing the number of hospital stays, and increasing patient and family comfort, the return on the investment is measured in both dollars and patient quality of life. This option promotes the idea that patient comfort and quality of life should be the priority when determining end-of-life care and planning.

What We Could Do

According to this option, we are not giving enough consideration to the quality of life of dying patients when considering treatment options. We need to make sure that patients have their desires recorded and honored when the time comes for administering end-of-life care. The overuse of invasive tests and procedures that degrade quality of life must be discontinued and more palliative options explored. Here are some actions this option suggests we take, along with some of their drawbacks:

■ **The American Medical Association and other governing boards should standardize a definition of "quality of life"** in a way that is universally understood. The criteria for determining "quality of life" should be critical in determining whether a procedure will be used.

■ **Hospitals, health insurance firms, and employers can require people to develop living wills** or advance directives. We would be able to decrease end-of-life suffering and unnecessary procedures.

■ **We should hold people accountable for their own quality of life.** Doctors should be able to withhold costly treatment and resources from those who make lifestyle choices that foster chronic illnesses. We waste too many resources on people who do not care enough to live better.

Trade-Offs and Downsides

■ **Everyone's personal definition of "quality of life"** is different. By allowing the medical boards to define this for us, we may be losing the ability to decide for ourselves what we want to do with our lives.

■ **People may change their minds.** At the time of developing a living will, people may feel they want treatment to stop at a certain point. However, in the moment of illness, they may want doctors to do all they can.

■ **It is unethical to withhold potentially lifesaving** interventions from people because a doctor does not like their life choices. It is not the doctor's place to judge people, only to help save lives.

Questions you might want to consider . . .

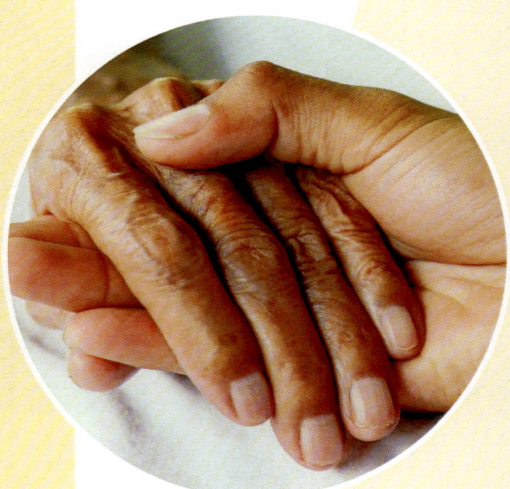

1 Imagine you are setting up a task force to establish standards for assessing quality of life of terminally ill patients. What voices should be represented in that group?

2 Some people are largely responsible for their own poor health. Do you think health-care professionals should refuse treatment—beyond comfort care—to seriously ill patients who persist in pursuing self-destructive lifestyles?

3 What palliative care options are available to terminally ill patients in your community? Are they accessible to everyone?

Option 2:
Preserve Life at All Costs

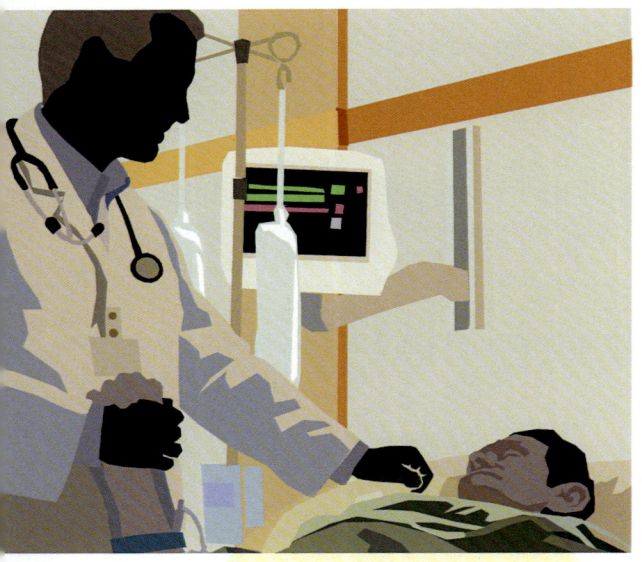

THIS OPTION HOLDS THAT ALL LIFE IS VALUABLE and always worth saving and that it is the obligation of society to preserve it by any means possible.

F. H. Epstein, of Harvard School of Medicine and Beth Israel Deaconess Medical Center, shares two stories illustrating this belief in *QJM*, an international medical journal. In one, the patient and physician adhered to the conviction that life should be preserved at all costs. In the second, a patient died "with dignity."

- A 45-year-old physician, blind and suffering from juvenile onset diabetes decided to end her life after three years of dialysis, but her physician convinced her to continue for one more month. That month proved to be a turning point. She began to learn Braille and became grateful to be alive. Within six months, her vision was restored and she eventually began working again.

- A 38-year-old homemaker with cervical cancer went through two years of radiation treatments before she was hospitalized with kidney failure, eventually becoming comatose. The attending physician said her cancer had spread. A close friend, with power of attorney, decided she had suffered enough and she was allowed to die. Her autopsy, however, showed that she did not have cancer. The problem was caused by an obstruction caused by the radiation treatments.

The homemaker may have lived decades longer had her doctor been required to do everything within his power, including seeking a second opinion. "The best way to ensure that a cure is not overlooked is to make it very hard for the physician to give up," Epstein writes. This option requires that medical doctors always go that extra mile to save lives.

Keeping patients alive may involve advanced medical treatments, participation in clinical trials, and even the use of life-support machines for those whose heart or lungs no longer work on their own. This option holds that such willingness to spend money on the dying shows our values as a nation. Even indigent people who have no resources have a right to the utmost in medical care.

Hold Doctors Ethically Accountable

Physicians take the Hippocratic Oath, swearing to "do no harm." Yet many reach the point in their medical careers in which their procedures and prescriptions risk injuring or killing patients. There may be no way to avoid this, but we can hold physicians ethically accountable for their decisions. Helping a patient hasten his or her own death is an injustice and a violation of the ancient role of the physician, according to this option, which views the application of medical knowledge for anything other than the promotion and sustenance of life as malpractice.

Writing in the *Journal of the American Medical Association*, Dr. David Graham, associate director of the US Office of Surveillance and Epidemiology, points out that "many modern oaths have a bland, generalized air of 'best wishes' about them, being near-meaningless formalities devoid of any influence on how medicine is truly practiced." But at one

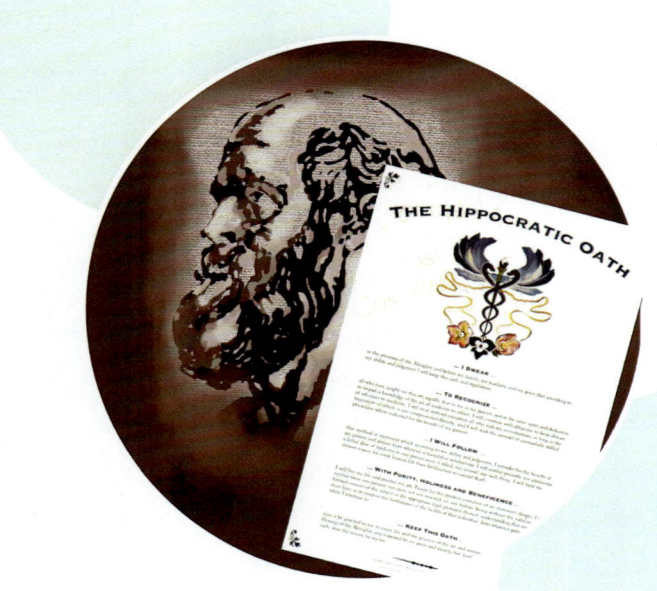

time, this was a binding document, outlining how physicians should morally conduct themselves.

"The reverence of each and every human life has been a keystone of Western medicine, and is the ethic which has caused physicians to try to preserve, protect, repair, prolong, and enhance every human life," according to Dr. J.P. Wilkie, writing in *California Medicine* in 1970.

According to this option, doctors should be held ethically and professionally accountable for the oath to "do no harm." Holding doctors accountable, by first ensuring all graduating medical doctors take the oath, and by making their oath professionally binding, will make it more difficult for them to do anything other than to try to preserve the lives of their patients as long as possible. Doctors who violate this oath should receive negative marks against their licenses, and their reputations should reflect this moral infraction.

Create Laws to Preserve Life

Passing laws is one way to ensure that medical doctors do all they can to preserve lives. The US Supreme Court supported this view almost 20 years ago. Justices ruled in favor of state laws that banned physician-assisted death, forcing doctors to maintain the life of a patient unless they had advance directives to the contrary. Before this ruling, doctors were allowed to use their own judgment, withdrawing or prolonging treatment at their discretion.

So far, 40 states have made medical aid in dying illegal. This option pushes for US courts to uphold these laws.

With this measure in place, we can help to minimize the number of people who die without every benefit of modern medicine's ability to prolong and sustain their lives decades beyond a negative prognosis. Valuing all life equally means that everyone would get the same care, even if the public has to pay for it.

Affirming the precious nature of life would also honor the religious traditions that many Americans cherish and with which they are comfortable.

Educate and Advocate

It is important for patients and family members to be informed and educated regarding end-of-life care options, according to the Family Care Alliance, an education and advocacy group for caregivers.

The more informed people are about their right to treatment, the more empowered they will be in the face of end-of-life decisions. "As a physician serving on our hospital ethics consult service, I find over 80 percent of our requests concern conflicting opinions between health care providers and patients' family members about when to transition to comfort care," wrote Dr. Deborah L. Kasman of Georgetown University's Department of Internal Medicine/Clinical Bioethics in the *Journal of General Internal Medicine*. "Discerning when medical interventions merely prolong dying is a distinctly modern challenge."

Educating families on treatment options and other aspects of end-of-life care can empower them to receive the treatment they desire and to hold doctors accountable. By leveling the playing field, education and advocacy serves the greater good and helps in the preservation of life for those facing terminal illnesses and traumatic situations.

Get a Second Opinion

In the United States, patients have certain legal rights when it comes to medical treatment. Advance directives are intended to inform health-care providers about the type of medical care an individual wants withheld—*or* provided—should they be unable to communicate their wishes.

©SUSAN M. GAETZ/GETTYIMAGES NEWS/GETTY IMAGES

Ellie Jenny and Brock Miller from the disability rights organization, Not Dead Yet, demonstrate against a court ruling upholding physician-assisted death.

QUESTIONNAIRE

End of Life:
What Should We Do for Those Who Are Dying?

You may also fill out this questionnaire online: www.nifi.org/questionnaires

NOW THAT YOU'VE HAD a chance to participate in a forum on this issue, we'd like to know what you're thinking. Anonymous responses will be included in summary reports on the forums and in research to help us better understand how people are thinking about current issues.

1. Do you agree or disagree with the statements below?

	Strongly Agree	Somewhat Agree	Somewhat Disagree	Strongly Disagree	Not Sure
a. Because life is sacred, a gift from God, we should do everything we can to preserve it.	☐	☐	☐	☐	☐
b. People who are terminally ill should have full control over how and when they die.	☐	☐	☐	☐	☐
c. Doctors should be more frank with patients and families about the pain and ultimate futility of many aggressive treatments for the terminally ill.	☐	☐	☐	☐	☐

QUESTIONNAIRE

(Question 2 continued from previous page)

	Strongly Favor	Somewhat Favor	Somewhat Oppose	Strongly Oppose	Not Sure
e. We should develop a network of "assisted dying" clinics to help terminal patients end their lives comfortably, EVEN IF that may make it easier for people who are depressed or temporarily losing hope to end their lives unnecessarily.	☐	☐	☐	☐	☐
f. Doctors should make every e ort to keep terminally ill patients alive for as long as possible, EVEN IF that involves ruinous expenses and, ultimately raises insurance rates for everyone.	☐	☐	☐	☐	☐

3. Are you thinking di erently about this issue now that you have participated in the forum?   ☐ Yes   ☐ No

If yes, how? _____

_____

_____

4. In your forum, did you talk about aspects of the issue you hadn't considered before?   ☐ Yes   ☐ No

If yes, please explain. _____

_____

6. Not including this forum, how many National Issues Forums have you attended?

☐ 0   ☐ 1-3   ☐ 4-6   ☐ 7 or more   ☐ Not sure

7. Are you male or female?   ☐ Male   ☐ Female

8. How old are you?

☐ 17 or younger   ☐ 18-30   ☐ 31-45   ☐ 46-64   ☐ 65 or older

9. Are you: ☐ African American   ☐ Asian American   ☐ Hispanic or Latino

☐ American Indian or Native American   ☐ White/Caucasian   ☐ Other (please specify) _____

10. Where do you live?   ☐ Rural   ☐ Small Town   ☐ Large City   ☐ Suburb

11. What is your ZIP code? _____   What state do you live in? _____

12. What issue would you like to see covered in a future forum? _____

Please give this form to the moderator, e-mail to forumreports@nifi.org, or mail to: National Issues Forums Institute, 100 Commons Road, Dayton, Ohio 45459.

You may also fill out this questionnaire online at www.nifi.org/questionnaires.

e. Insurance companies, hospitals, and other health-care facilities should require all their clients to make living wills.

f. Helping a patient die is a violation of the oath all doctors take to "do no harm."

2. Do you favor or oppose each of these actions?

	Strongly Favor	Somewhat Favor	Somewhat Oppose	Strongly Oppose	Not Sure
a. We should make physician-assisted death legal in all 50 states, EVEN IF that means some patients may feel pressured to choose death as a way to relieve the burden on their families.	☐	☐	☐	☐	☐
b. Doctors should not be subject to malpractice suits for withholding aggressive treatment of terminally ill patients if such treatment will cause more su ering, EVEN IF there is a chance it would prolong the patient's life long enough to find a cure.	☐	☐	☐	☐	☐
c. Government and private insurers should invest more money into hospice care, EVEN IF that would divert funds from prevention and treatment programs.	☐	☐	☐	☐	☐
d. We should roll back state laws that legalize physician-assisted death, EVEN IF this takes away the ability of people to control their own lives.	☐	☐	☐	☐	☐

(Question 2 continued on next page)

But numerous agencies, including the National Academy of Elder Law Attorneys, have found that implementation of advance directives varies greatly from state to state. The National Right to Life Committee reported that the laws of 21 states and territories "provide no effective protection of a patient's wishes for life-preserving measures in the face of an unwilling health-care provider."

Thus, it is essential, in this view, that doctors who insist on withdrawing treatment or who determine the point of medical futility should be required to consult with other health-care providers who are not directly involved with the patient. This will allow for unbiased second opinions and increase the potential for discovering viable options for sustaining patient lives.

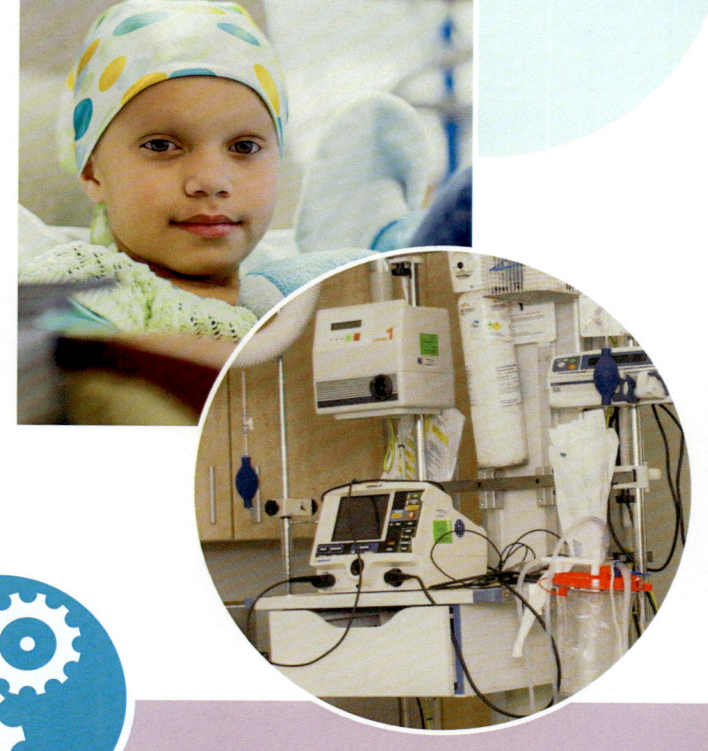

What We Could Do

This option takes the view that our first priority is preserving life at all costs. With advances in medical technology, we are fully capable of sustaining and prolonging life in the face of terminal illnesses. We must do everything possible to ensure that health-care providers are not cutting corners and refusing life-extending treatments to those who are dying. This is both the legal and moral thing to do. Here are some actions supported by this option.

■ **We could educate families and patients regarding their legal rights** to demand treatment and to require doctors to sustain their lives at all costs.

■ **We can force doctors to participate in peer consultations** with health-care professionals not directly involved with their patients. This will provide an unbiased opinion regarding the direction that end-of-life care should go, and thus, make it more difficult for doctors to "give up."

■ **We could appeal to the Supreme Court to roll back all state laws that have legalized physician-assisted death.** This will return our nation to its previous state of preserving the rights of every citizen, especially their right to live.

Trade-Offs and Downsides

■ **This approach may unnecessarily create combative patients** and families who are too willing to fight health-care professionals who are clearly more qualified to make medical decisions than the patient and family.

■ **This would add more duties to health-care professionals** already inundated by heavy caseloads. It could also add an enormous expense to what is already the world's most expensive health-care system.

■ **This could weaken the sovereignty of individual state governments** and thereby reduce people's faith in their elected officials and the democratic process. To roll back state laws is to clearly undermine the authority of states and the wishes of their people.

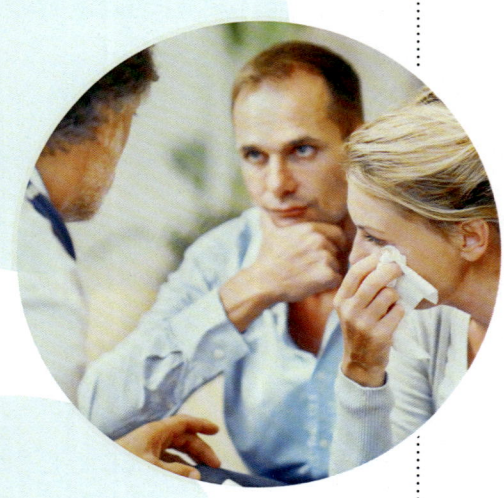

Questions you might want to consider . . .

1 Could a case be made that, under some circumstances, keeping a suffering patient alive is actually dishonoring the Hippocratic Oath to "do no harm"?

2 What might be the consequences for allowing doctors to prescribe drugs to help patients die?

3 As medical science continues to advance, what, if any, limits should be placed on how long, and under what conditions, dying patients should be kept alive?

Option 3:
My Right, My Choice

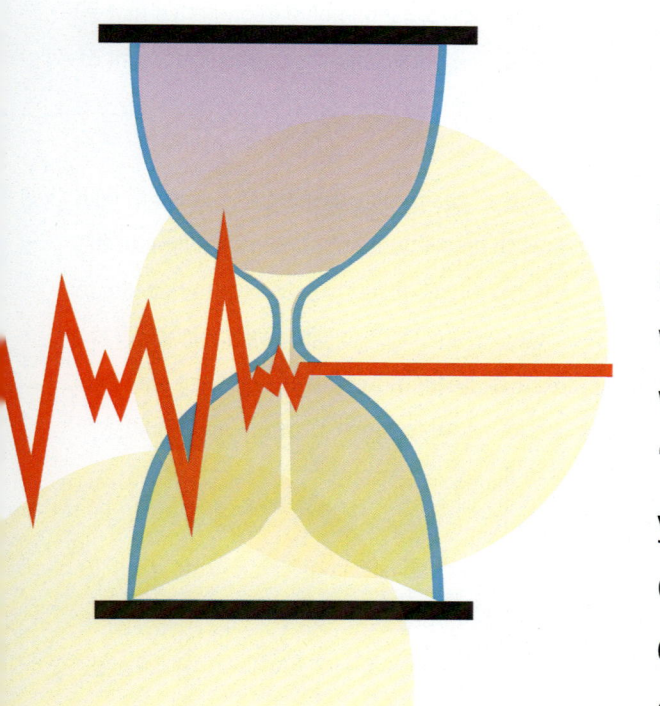

KAREN ANN QUINLAN WAS ONLY 21 years old in 1975 when she collapsed into a coma from which she could never recover. Though treatment was ended a year later, she continued living in a "persistent vegetative state" for almost 10 more years before dying of pneumonia. At the time of her death, she weighed 65 pounds. Quinlan's case, which made coast-to-coast headlines, is credited with fueling the right-to-die movement.

Some 30 years later, in 2016, California became the 5th state to pass right-to-die legislation. The new law brought considerable peace of mind to terminally ill cancer patient Kristy Allan, who had exhausted all viable chemotherapy options. The 63-year-old told NBC News she felt she had taken control of how she wanted to live by choosing to stop further treatment, and now she was also able to take some control over how she wanted to die.

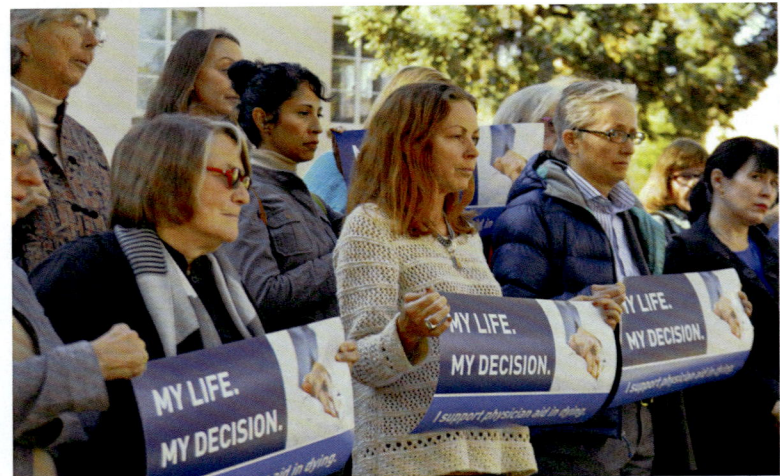

©AP PHOTO/RUSSELL CONTRERAS

"What we're doing should be available to any patient with an incurable, horrible disease that they've tried everything on, and it doesn't seem to work," Dr. Lawrence Egbert, whose license was suspended in Maryland for assisting in six patient deaths, told the *New York Times*.

Not everyone chooses to end life. Doctors said 15-year-old Jahi McMath was brain dead after surgery in 2013. Her family refused to remove her from life support and two years later, stood by the decision to keep her alive.

Performing surgeries and other complex and expensive procedures on those with no hope for a cure, only inflicts unnecessary physical and financial burdens on patients who otherwise would rather just die in peace. But withholding treatment when a patient desires it is equally wrong. According to this option, everyone should have the right to choose.

Legalize Right-to-Die in All States

As of early 2016, only Oregon, California, Montana, Vermont, and Washington have authorized death-with-dignity practices. In this view, the slow movement towards legalization of physician-assisted death is nothing but a hindrance to people who need the right to choose. It puts more people at risk, forcing them to find dangerous and unregulated ways to take their own lives.

This option holds that all states should legalize the freedom to choose, giving people the liberty to determine their life paths. A May 2013 Gallup poll demonstrated that 70 percent of Americans supported the use and development of end-of-life initiatives, yet it has remained illegal in 90 percent of states.

Without universal legalization, dying people have to take extreme measures to die without suffering. In addition to the stress of being terminally ill, patients may have to relocate to one of the few states where right-to-die laws are in effect in order to exercise their freedom to choose. This just isn't fair to those who cannot afford to move, or who are too physically debilitated to do so.

Every US citizen should have the same access to this right to choose. Legalizing physician-assisted death in all 50 states and the District of Columbia would bring equality and justice, while showing compassion for those who are dying.

Standardize Right-to-Die Protocols

People have found many creative, and sometimes dangerous, ways to end their lives. Some stop eating and drinking, while others inhale carbon monoxide or take various drugs. Without standardization, people are left to experiment. Many medical procedures are standardized. Why not the process of dying by choice?

Advocacy groups like the Right to Die Network, Final Exit Network, and Compassion and Choices support the right to die for people suffering from terminal illnesses. Barbara Coombs Lee, president of Compassion and Choices, supports the use of doctor-prescribed medications for ending one's life. But not everyone who receives them will use them. "They want to have it the same way you want an umbrella or you want fire insurance or you want a safety blanket of some kind," she told CNN. It's about having the option.

This option says that people who choose to end their lives should be able to do so without stigma and without the risks of further harming themselves by using dangerous and nonstandardized methods. It's about safety and informed decision making.

Understand the Options

Education is empowering. Empowering dying patients can help reduce feelings of helplessness and depression, two factors that contribute to the numbers of those requesting to end their lives. Some sources report that close to 60 percent of practicing physicians have received such requests. Although difficult, these requests open opportunities for physicians to discuss the existing options and their consequences.

But it's not totally up to doctors. Many groups serve to educate people dealing with end-of-life choices. Outlined in the EPEC (Educating Physicians on End-of-Life Care) Participant's Handbook is a six-step process for responding to a patient's request to hasten death. These steps provide a protocol for educating both the physician and the patient.

This option holds that patients should have every opportunity to choose life or

death when facing a terminal illness. This decision is best exercised when patients are well informed about the risks and outcomes of their choices.

Create Death-with-Dignity Laws in the United States

Four states currently have statutes that allow mentally competent, terminally ill patients with six or fewer months to live, to opt for "death with dignity." Laws in these states allow physicians to prescribe drugs, which patients may choose to take when or if they are no longer willing to endure the pain and suffering that lies between them and imminent death.

All of these laws include a variety of protections designed to safeguard patients and prevent misuse. Two physicians must confirm that the patient's condition is imminently terminal, that he or she is mentally competent, and that the request for the lethal drug has been made

States that Authorized Death-with-Dignity Practices by the End of 2015

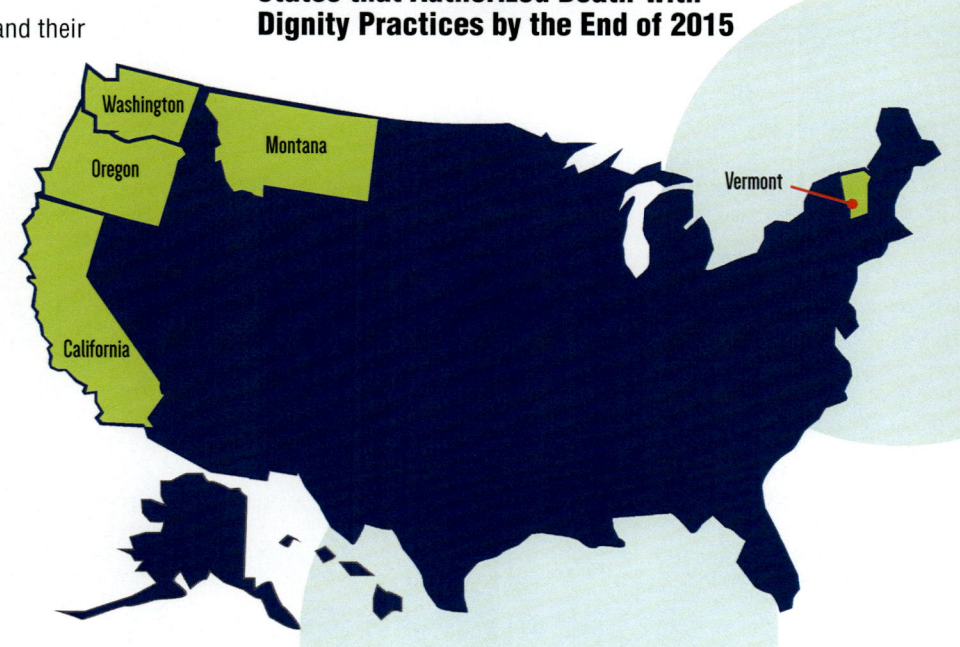

voluntarily. In Oregon, the patient must make two separate requests for the medication, separated by at least 15 days; in addition, a 48-hour waiting period is mandated between the time the patient receives the prescription and has it filled.

All these laws stipulate that only the patient—not a doctor and not a friend or family member—may administer the lethal medication. And, in fact, armed with the power to make their own choices, many patients do not, in the end, exercise it. In the first 10 years in Oregon, only about 65 percent of such patients actually used the lethal prescriptions.

Montana does not currently have a death-with-dignity law on the books, but the procedure is legal in that state by judicial fiat. In 2009, the state's Supreme Court ruled that nothing in the state laws prohibits a physician from writing a prescription for a lethal drug requested by a mentally competent, terminally ill patient who wants to hasten death.

Remove Legal Penalties for Doctors Who Assist

Legal or illegal, a number of physicians have reported honoring a patient's request to die. According to a recent study, 4.7 percent of physicians admitted to giving lethal injections to kill suffering patients upon request (honoring 54 percent of requests). By doing so, physicians risk having their licenses revoked and being subjected to criminal charges.

Why should doctors be penalized for fulfilling a patient's request to end his or her suffering? As long as a physician is acting in good faith, there should be no legal consequences. According to this option, physician-assisted death should be legalized in every state and all legal penalties should be overturned. Patients choosing to exercise this right should be given information and support services to assist their decision making and provide peace of mind to their loved ones.

What We Could Do

This option is concerned that stiff legal penalties and the small number of states that have legalized physician-assisted deaths unfairly burden many Americans and deprive them of their right to choose how they will die. This only encourages the use of dangerous procedures by patients who wish to die with dignity and can't get help. Here are some things this option suggests we should do, along with some drawbacks:

■ **The federal government should legalize physician-assisted death** in all 50 states and the District of Columbia. Leaving it as a state-by-state decision unfairly burdens the majority of the population.

■ **The American Medical Association should work to standardize protocols for physician-assisted deaths,** making it unnecessary for people to come up with their own ways of taking their own lives.

■ **Health-care professionals should be absolved of all legal penalties** for assisting in the death of patients. Medical doctors who have been penalized should have their penalties reversed and their professional status restored.

Trade-Offs and Downsides

■ **To impose such a law on individual states undermines and weakens** their autonomy and could create discord between federal and state governments. Such "big brother" authority erodes democracy.

■ **Not everyone will be able to afford the standardized methods** and people will continue to find alternative methods for ending their lives. By developing a standard approach, the AMA will be supporting people who commit suicide. And having such standard protocols in place may make the decision to die seem as commonplace as any other medical procedure.

■ **Without the threat of legal sanctions,** some health-care professionals may abuse the lack of oversight, and pressure members of underserved populations to unnecessarily take their lives. The medical code of ethics will become a joke.

Questions you might want to consider . . .

1 What, if any, legal limits should be placed on the right of a physician to help an adult patient with a terminal disease choose death, if that is the patient's wish?

2 In places where physician-assisted death is legal, would you favor the development of so-called "assisted-dying" clinics," such as those found in Switzerland? What might be the advantages and drawbacks?

3 Should parents be allowed to make the decision to seek physician-assisted death for minor children in the last stages of a debilitating terminal disease?

Summary

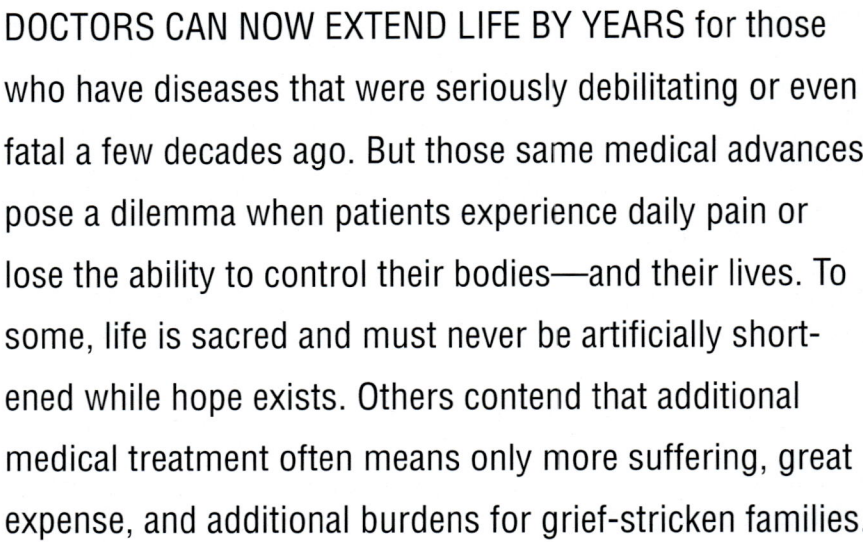

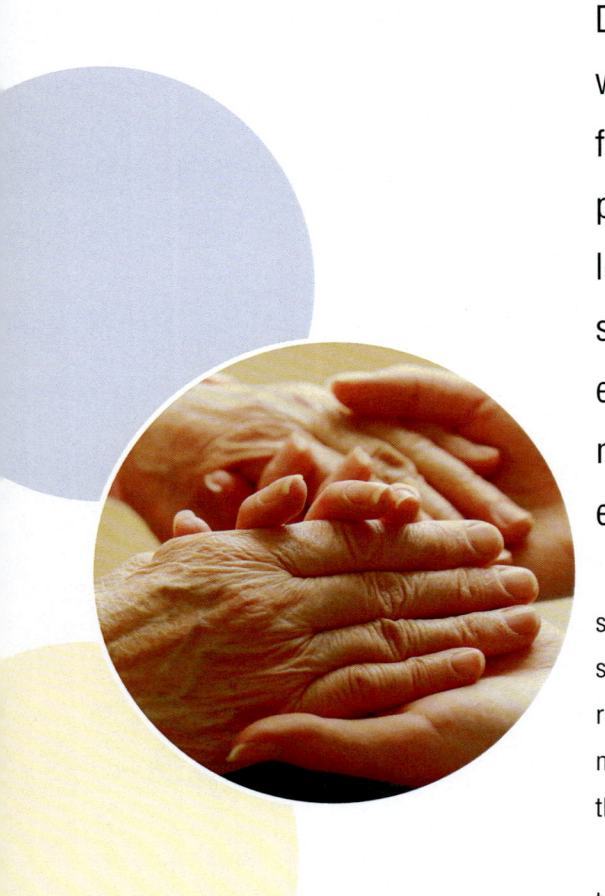

DOCTORS CAN NOW EXTEND LIFE BY YEARS for those who have diseases that were seriously debilitating or even fatal a few decades ago. But those same medical advances pose a dilemma when patients experience daily pain or lose the ability to control their bodies—and their lives. To some, life is sacred and must never be artificially shortened while hope exists. Others contend that additional medical treatment often means only more suffering, great expense, and additional burdens for grief-stricken families.

A growing "death with dignity" movement is reflected in the laws of several states that allow physician-assisted death. Doctors in these and many other states take less active steps simply by withholding draconian treatments at the request of patients and their families. Others say that legalizing any of these measures will cheapen life and make it too easy to prematurely end the lives of the terminally ill.

While we will not all have to grapple with decisions about medical care for a terminally ill family member, we all subsidize that care through our tax dollars and insurance premiums. The question is, at the end of life, who should decide how or when we die?

Option 1:

Maintain Quality of Life

MEDICAL ADVANCES MAKE IT POSSIBLE to keep people alive long after they might otherwise have died naturally. People should be able to opt for discontinuing treatment when prolonging life promises only further pain and suffering. Doctors should focus on the quality of the lives of terminally ill patients in their care.

EXAMPLES OF WHAT SHOULD BE DONE	TRADE-OFFS TO CONSIDER
Doctors should be required to employ the least invasive and least harmful treatments for terminal diseases.	This will limit doctors and may mean that some people will not get the aggressive treatment that they may wish.
The AMA and governing medical boards should develop, adopt, and mandate certain standards regarding quality of life.	People may not agree with the standards that professional boards believe represent quality of life, and certain voices may be left out of the conversation.
Hospitals and health insurance companies should require living wills that clearly spell out "terms of death" for anyone with a terminal illness.	People change their minds. To force individuals to create living wills may lock them into agreements that may or may not reflect their true intentions. The pressure may influence the terms.
Lifestyle choices should be taken into consideration in selecting treatment for terminal illnesses. Late-stage alcoholics, for example, should not be eligible for scarce and costly liver transplants.	Often, the choices we make are influenced by inherited traits or our environment. In addition, some people who are addicted may not have had access to treatment to help them stop.
What else?	What's the trade-off?

Option 2:
Preserve Life at All Costs

THOSE DRAWN TO THIS OPTION feel it is the obligation of society to preserve life at all costs regardless of patients' wishes and those of their families. All life is valuable and worth saving. We have a collective moral responsibility to do everything possible to prevent death. As long as there is the ability to maintain life, our skills should be employed in sustaining it.

EXAMPLES OF WHAT SHOULD BE DONE

TRADE-OFFS TO CONSIDER

EXAMPLES OF WHAT SHOULD BE DONE	TRADE-OFFS TO CONSIDER
Ethically, doctors should make every effort to keep patients alive. It's a part of their oath to do no harm.	This could result in a great deal of unnecessary suffering and high medical costs. Not all patients would want their lives prolonged.
Lawmakers should make it mandatory for doctors to provide all available options to sustain an individual's life, regardless of prognosis.	This would violate individual freedom because it would allow public officials to interfere with people's medical care.
Advocacy groups should educate families and patients about their medical options and their right to treatment.	Such groups could interfere with the wishes of patients and their families. This could also keep families from accepting terminal diagnoses.
End-of-life treatment decisions should involve consultations with doctors not directly involved with the patient to get a second, unbiased opinion.	This could be expensive and time-consuming. Some patients would not want to consult with doctors they do not know.
What else?	What's the trade-off?

Option 3:

My Right, My Choice

THE FREEDOM TO CHOOSE FOR ONESELF, as long as it does not directly infringe upon the rights of others, is a deeply held American value. People should all have the right to decide whether they want to live or die. We should expand the options available to all of us at the end of our lives to include the right to seek help from our physicians in ending our lives when death is inevitable and suffering makes life unendurable.

EXAMPLES OF WHAT SHOULD BE DONE	TRADE-OFFS TO CONSIDER
Government should legally grant people the freedom to determine when and how they want to die.	This could burden families and encourage an increase in impulsive acts of suicide. People with mental illness, such as depression, may be particularly at risk.
The medical profession should develop standard and systematic means to assist patients in ending life in ways that are both successful and humane.	This may trivialize death by making it seem like an easy choice.
Schools and advocacy groups could educate citizens regarding the impact of death on society and families so they can make more informed decisions about living or dying.	People suffering the physical and emotional effects of a terminal illness may not be in any state to make rational, "educated" decisions.
Create clinics where people can go to receive assistance with dying.	Such clinics could easily lead to killing people unnecessarily.
What else?	What's the trade-off?

The National Issues Forums

The National Issues Forums (NIF) is a network of organizations that brings together citizens around the nation to talk about pressing social and political issues of the day. Thousands of community organizations, including schools, libraries, churches, civic groups, and others, have sponsored forums designed to give people a public voice in the affairs of their communities and their nation.

Forum participants engage in deliberation, which is simply weighing options for action against things held commonly valuable. This calls upon them to listen respectfully to others, sort out their views in terms of what they most value, consider courses of action and their disadvantages, and seek to identify actionable areas of common ground.

Issue guides like this one are designed to frame and support these deliberations. They present varying perspectives on the issue at hand, suggest actions to address identified problems, and note the trade-offs of taking those actions to remind participants that all solutions have costs as well as benefits.

In this way, forum participants move from holding individual opinions to making collective choices as members of a community—the kinds of choices from which public policy may be forged or public action may be taken, on community as well as national levels.

Feedback

If you participated in this forum, please fill out a questionnaire, which is included in this issue guide or can be accessed online at **www.nifi.org/questionnaires**. If you are filling out the enclosed questionnaire, please return the completed form to your moderator or to the National Issues Forums Institute, 100 Commons Road, Dayton, Ohio 45459.

If you moderated this forum, please fill out a Moderator Response sheet, which is online at **www.nifi.org/questionnaires**.

Your responses play a vital role in providing information that is used to communicate your views to others, including officeholders, the media, and other citizens.